YOUR GUIDE FOR A HEALTHY

LIFE

2nd

EDITION

BY

KIBOKO FRANÇOISE MACHOZI

www.savelife.co.za

CONTENTS

5

This health booklet is made with a purpose of helping you to understand your condition, to prevent and to discover diseases from the beginning, but it must not replace your doctor's consultation and instructions.
If by reading it you discover that you are sick, please consult your doctor and follow his or her instructions.
Do not forget that self-medication can kill you or worsen your condition.

INTRODUCTION

This manual is made with a purpose of helping you to know about your health and how to take care not only of yourself but also your families.

It is difficult for an individual to take a doctor's instruction, if he does not understand the reason. Most of the time the doctors have long queues and do not have enough time to explain properly to the patients the reason for their instructions, and even when they do people may forget.

Health is priceless; to maintain it, we need sufficient knowledge. We learn through circumstances, from a speech or from a book. I am always amazed when I receive an invitation to give a health speech, but this time I think writing a health booklet will be much more beneficial than just giving a speech. In French we say, "*Les paroles s'en volent mais les écrits restent.*" This means, people forget what they hear, but a book will always be there as a reminder. A speech will attend to a limited community, but a book will go far.

When we learn through circumstances, it is difficult to forget the experience, but in health matters we must not wait for a person to be sick so that we may learn, because it may be too late; that is the reason why we say that "prevention is better than a cure"

1. HEALTH

The word *health* has been discussed in the dictionary[i].

"Health is the state of an organism when it functions optimally, without evidence of disease or abnormality: A state characterized by anatomic, physiologic, and psychological integrity; ability to perform personally valued family, work, and community roles; ability to deal with physical, biological, psychological, and social stress; a feeling of well-being; and freedom from the risk of disease and untimely death. Complete physical, mental, and social wellbeing, not just the absence of disease, as defined by the World Health Organization."

2. HUMAN DEVELOPMENT

Both men and women develop and pass through different stages, per the discussions to follow.

CHILDHOOD

Childhood starts from birth until eight years of age, but the length of this period varies from one child to another. For some children, especially boys, it may last up to eleven or twelve years of age.

REPRODUCTIVE PERIOD

This period starts at puberty and, for women, ends at menopause. During this period a woman is able to conceive and bear a child. A man is able to impregnate. The reproductive period concerns two different periods: puberty and adult age.

PUBERTY

"Puberty is a sequence of events by which a child becomes a young adult, characterized by the beginning of female or male sex cells, secretion of sexual hormones, and development of secondary sexual characteristics and reproductive functions; sexual dimorphism (difference in the appearance between girls and boys) is accentuated. In girls the first sign of puberty may be evident at the age of eight years, with the process largely completed by age sixteen; in boys puberty commonly begins at ages ten to twelve and is largely completed at age eighteen.

Ethnic and geographic factors may influence the time at which various events typical of puberty occur".[ii]

Per example a study done in America show that African Americans present the first signs of puberty earlier than white Americans.[iii]

ADULT

"An adult is a living organism that has attained full growth or maturity".[iv]

MENOPAUSE

"Menopause is the permanent cessation of the menses or menstrual life".[v]

3. NUTRITION AND DIET

NUTRIENTS GROUPS

There are four groups of nutrients, as discussed below.

PROTEINS

Proteins are nutrients that build up body cells of human beings. There are two different types of proteins:

• Animal proteins: e.g., meat, fish, eggs, dairy products

• Vegetable proteins: e.g., beans, lentils, soya, peanuts

Children need ten grams of proteins per day
Teenagers' boys need fifty-two grams of proteins per day
Teenagers' girls need forty-six grams of proteins per day
Adult men need fifty-six grams of proteins per day

Adult women need forty-six grams of proteins per day and pregnant women need seventy-one grams of protein per day.[vi]

NB: Excessive amounts (more than what an individual of a certain age or weight with a particular physical activity suppose to take per day)of protein are dangerous for kidneys.

CARBOHYDRATES AND LIPIDS

Carbohydrates and lipids are foods that give you energy.

Carbohydrates are subdivided into two subgroups:

• Cereals (e.g., rice, maize, wheat, barley, oat, rye, millet, and buckwheat)

• Vegetables (e.g., cassava, potatoes, Hubbard squashes, banana, pumpkins, caladium, butternuts, and taro root)

Lipids or fat

Examples of lipids or fats include oil, margarine, and dairy products.

VITAMINS AND MINERALS

Vitamins are organic elements produced by plants and animals; they are sensitive to light, heat, air, and acid. Minerals are inorganic elements found in water and in soil. They are absorbed by plants. Minerals do not change their natural structure despite the environmental conditions. Vitamins and minerals help in metabolic reactions. They act as antioxidants, catalysts, coenzymes, and as cell-regulation mediators. They promote tissue differentiation and tissue growth, convert sugar into energy, promote proteins and fatty acids synthesis, and boost the immune system.[vii]

When we eat food, our bodies do not use food the way we eat it. There is gastric juice and some saprophyte germs found in the

digestive tract (such as *Entamoeba coli*) that do not harm the body but help to break down the molecules of the food we eat. Vitamins and minerals help in the process of building up new molecules that are useful for our bodies; this reaction also leads to the emergence of free radicals that damage cells and harm the body.

NB: Free radicals may also be created by the following:

The immune system (in the process of fighting infections).

Tobacco smoke, air pollution, herbicides, and radiations.

Among vitamins and minerals, we find other elements that neutralize free radicals. We call them antioxidants.[viii]

What is a free radical, and what is an antioxidant?

A free radical or ion is a molecule that has fewer than eight electrons on its last shell, or a molecule that has lost one or some of its electrons and becomes unstable, looking for electrons to steal so it may be stable.

Oxidation is a process whereby a molecule releases its own electrons to another molecule. In such a case, a stable molecule may also release some of its electrons to stabilize a free radical.

The molecule releasing electrons becomes a free radical and starts to seek stability by taking electrons from other molecules. This may lead to the destruction of cells and emergence of diseases.

An antioxidant is a molecule that inhibits the oxidation of other molecules by releasing its own electrons to stabilize free radicals.[ix]

Reaction antioxidant and free radicals

An atom is composed of a nucleus that is surrounded by shells.

In an atom's nucleus, we find positively charged particles called protons.

Shells are filled in by negatively charged particles called electrons. For an atom to be stable, the total number of electrons on shells must be equal to the number of protons in the atom's nucleus.

In a case that the number of electrons on shells becomes lesser or higher than the number of protons in the atom's nucleus, this atom will be called an ion and it will try to stabilize itself by different ways:

1. By stealing electrons from the nearest stable atom, this process may cause cell damage and the emergence of several diseases. In such a case, the presence of an antioxidant may solve the problem, because

the antioxidant will prevent the oxidation of other molecules by releasing its own electrons to the ion or free radical.

2. By sharing its own electrons with other free radicals.

NB: Electrons unite atoms to make molecules and unite molecules to make cells.

Cells constitute a human's body.

3. By giving to another free radical electrons found on its outer shell.[x]

Some antioxidants and their sources

VITAMIN A

There are two different kinds of vitamin A:

1. Preformed vitamin A or retinal, found in animal liver, dairy products, and egg yolks.

2. Provitamin A or beta-carotene, found in plants.

Sources of beta-carotene:

Sweet potatoes

Carrots

Mangoes

Spinach

Dried apricots

VITAMIN B2 (Riboflavin)

Sources

Almond, eggs, milk, yogurt, organ meat, whole grain, wheat germ, wild rice, mushrooms, soy beans, brussels sprouts, broccoli, sprouts, and spinach

VITAMIN C (Ascorbic acid)

Sources

Lemon, oranges, mandarins (*naarties*)

VITAMIN E (Alpha-tocopherol)

Sources

Beef liver

Fortified cereals, nuts, and seeds

Wheat germ

Peanuts

Margarine

Vegetable oil

Green vegetables

Papaya

Olives

LYCOPENE

Sources

Tomatoes

Watermelon

Pink grapefruit

Pink guava

Papaya

Apricots

Rose hip

SELENIUM

Sources

Spinach

Corn

Brazil nuts

Garlic

Sunflower seed

Salmon

Meat

Tuna

Calf's liver

FIBERS

Fibers are hard parts of plants that are not digested by gastrointestinal enzymes until they reach the colon. The main role of fibers is to maintain the digestive tract, so it may work efficiently.

There are two different kinds of fibers: soluble and insoluble. Soluble fibers absorb water and form a sort of gel that delays digestion, the fact of delaying digestion decreases your appetite, helps you to control your weight, affects glucose absorption, increases insulin sensitivity, and controls diabetes mellitus. Soluble fibers bind themselves to the bile acid and decrease fat's absorption. In the colon, bacteria ferment soluble fibers into gases.

Insoluble fibers do not absorb water but release all the waste and toxins, as they may lead to several diseases. Insoluble fibers have a laxative effect and prevent constipation. They promote the growth of bacteria that ferment and soften the waste.

High-fiber foods help to maintain normal blood sugar and prevent constipation, hemorrhoids, colon cancer, heart disease, and much more. We find a considerable amount of fiber in fresh and dry fruits, grains, beans, nuts, seeds, legumes, and vegetables.[xi]

Some foods rich in soluble fibers

Oatmeal, oat cereals, carrots, strawberries, blueberries, celery, oranges, apples, pears, nuts, cucumber, beans, lentils, and flaxseeds.

Some foods rich in insoluble fibers

Whole grain, whole wheat, wheat bran, corn bran, couscous, seeds, nuts, brown rice, barley, green beans, raisins, grapefruits, carrots, bulgur, cucumber, zucchini, tomatoes, onions, celery, cabbages, dark and leafy vegetables, and root vegetable's skin.[xii]

For an illustration

When you want to make a cake, you need the following: Flour, eggs, and sugar, which come from wheat, sugarcane, and chicken, respectively.

To make wheat into flour, we need a grinding machine.

To make sugarcane into sugar, we also need a   special   process.

To blend the eggs, we do need a mixer . When you have the flour, sugar, and eggs, you can bake a cake.

In our bodies, when we eat any food, we need the gastric juice; we also need those saprophyte germs to break down whatever we eat.

To bake a cake we need a blender to mix up flour, eggs, and sugar; we also need a bowl and an oven to bake our cake.

After the gastric juice and saprophyte germs have finished breaking down eaten food, our bodies need vitamins and minerals to build up new molecules that are useful for the body.

In the same way, after baking our cake, we need to clean up the dirt from the food we cooked, so our bodies need fibers to clean up all the toxins and waste remaining from the digestion process.

Everybody needs a balanced meal: that is, a meal that consists of all the food from the basic food groups of nutrients (but, depending on their ages, different people will express different preferences).

Children need more proteins to build up their bodies. This does not mean that other groups are not important; they are still important but not like proteins, because the child is still in a period where he or she is busy building up body and brain.

Avoid giving your children saturated fats and chemically rich sugar-foods and -drinks, but encourage them to drink enough water and help them to be physically active.

Teenagers need more food that gives energy, but they have to limit their intake of fats and chemically rich sugar-foods and drinks.

They have to eat plenty of vegetables and fruits. A portion of proteins big as the palm of a teenager's hand (forty-two to fifty-two grams) two times per day is enough. [xiii]They have to drink plenty of water and exercise on a regular basis.

Adults need more vitamins and minerals.

Also, adults still need proteins and carbohydrates, but they have to limit their intake of saturated fats, salt, chemically rich sugar-foods and -drinks. Adults have to drink plenty of water and exercise on a regular basis.

MALNUTRITION

In this chapter, we will concentrate on three different forms of nutritional problems: undernourishment, obesity and high cholesterol

UNDERNOURISHMENT

This happens most of the time to children. There are many kinds of undernourishment problems, some of which are discussed below:

1. MARASMUS

"Marasmus is a form of protein-caloric chiefly occurring during the first year of life, characterized by growth retardation and progressive wasting of subcutaneous fat and muscle, but usually with retention of the appetite and mental alertness. Infectious diseases may be precipitating factors. Marasmus is now considered to be related to kwashiorkor, also called infantile atrophy, trepsiapedatrophy, and decomposition

(Finkelstein), *M. infantilis*, and *M. lactanium.*"[xiv]

2. KWASHIORKOR

"Kwashiorkor syndrome is produced by severe protein deficiency, characterized by retarded growth, changes in skin and hair pigment, edema, and pathologic changes in the liver, including fatty infiltration, necrosis, and fibrosis. Other findings are peevish mental apathy, atrophy of the pancreas, gastrointestinal disorder, anemia, low serum albumin, and dermatoses. The skin may exhibit dark, thickened patches on limbs and back, which may desquamate or peel off in scales, leaving a pink, almost raw surface of a pellagroid (condition characterized by diarrhea, dementia and dermatitis due to a vitamin deficiency) appearance. First reported from Africa, kwashiorkor is now known to occur throughout the world, but mainly in the tropics and subtropics, and is now considered to be related to marasmus.

Marasmic kwashiorkor: A condition in which there is deficiency of both calories and proteins, with severe tissue wasting, loss of subcutaneous fat, and usually dehydration."[xv]

3. AVITAMINOSIS

Avitaminosis is defined as a lack or insufficiency of some vitamins. It may be caused by a diet poor in a specific vitamin: for example a person taking a diet poor in vitamin B1 (Thiamine) may develop Beriberi. It may be also caused by a deficit in the metabolic conversion of some vitamins: for example elderly kidneys are less able to convert vitamin D to its active form as consequence their risk of developing vitamin D deficiency is high and they end up developing osteomalacia. Avitaminosis may also be the consequence of some diseases: for example a person suffering from Thyphoid to whom a big portion of small intestine has been removed may present vitamin B12 deficiency (megaloblastic anemia) as this specific vitamin is absorbed in the last portion of the small intestine.

Some diseases are caused by a long-term vitamin deficiency: for example deficiency in vitamin C causes scurvy.

Some vitamins, and their roles, sources and deficiency

1. VITAMIN A is an antioxidant; it plays an important role in the growth and repair of body cells and promotes good sight, healthy skin, and healthy bones and teeth formation.

Source

- Animal liver
- Milk
- Egg yolks
- Sweet potatoes
- Carrots
- Mangoes
- Spinach
- Dried apricots

Vitamin A deficiency causes *xerophtalmia* or night blindness or dry-eye syndrome. The deficiency may itself be caused by alcohol, coffee, and irons that may disturb body absorption of vitamin A.

2. Vitamin B1 or thiamine is very important for neurological, organ, and cellular function.

Sources of vitamin B1 or thiamine

- Sunflower seeds

- Sesame butter

- Coriander leaves

- Poppy seeds

- Mustard seeds

- Paprika

- Rosemary

- Thyme

- Pistachio nuts

- Macadamia nuts

- Pecan nuts

- Fish

Deficiency in thiamine or vitamin B1 causes *beriberi*, which is a disease characterized by cardiovascular abnormalities and neurological and gastrointestinal troubles.

3. Vitamin B2 or riboflavin acts as an antioxidant.

It converts carbohydrates into glucose, which is burned up to produce energy. It prevents cataract and eye lens damage. It promotes good sight, healthy eyes, healthy skin, hair growth, a healthy liver, fats and proteins' metabolism, red blood cells synthesis and body growth.

Vitamin B2 helps the nervous system to work properly. It converts vitamin B6 and folic acid into their useful form. It also decreases the number of migraine attacks.

Sources of Riboflavin

Almond, yogurt, milk, eggs, organ meats, whole grains, wheat germ, wild rice, soy beans, brussels sprouts, broccoli, mushrooms, sprout and spinach.

Riboflavin deficiency causes digestive troubles, colored tongue, sores on mouth corners, sore throat, fatigue, slowed growth, edema, sensitivity to light, and eye fatigue.

4. Vitamin B3 or niacin is an important cellular nutrient; it breaks down carbohydrates and lipids in order to produce energy, it breaks down proteins in order to build up cells. Vitamin B3 is very important for the maintenance of good mental and neurological function.

Vitamin B3 promotes good blood circulation, decreases the level of cholesterol, and promotes hormonal synthesis, as well as acting as an antioxidant. Vitamin B3 is also used to treat arthritis.

Sources of vitamin B3 or niacin

• Peanuts

• Sesame seeds

• Sunflower seeds

• Wheat germ

• Avocado

• Mushrooms

• Cereals

• Fish

• Peas

Vitamin B3 deficiency causes *pellagra,* which is a condition characterized by nausea, vomiting, balance disorder, seizures, fatigue, headache, dermatologic disorders, diarrhea, and depression, and, if it is not treated, it may lead to death.

Causes of Vitamin B3 deficiency

Vitamin B3 deficiency is caused by the following:

• The intake of no diversified foods.

• Alcoholism

• Some diseases, such as

    diabetes mellitus,

    intestinal cancer,

    liver cirrhosis, and

    hyperthyroidism.

5. Vitamin B5, or pantothenic acid, is useful for energy production, synthesis of acetylcholine (useful chemical for the nervous system and the heart), steroidal hormones, vitamin A, vitamin D, fatty acids, and cholesterol metabolism. Sources of vitamin B5 include egg yolk and fresh vegetables. Deficiency in pantothenic acid causes *fatigue*.

6. Vitamin B6 or pyridoxine regulates the activity of the nervous system and promotes sugar metabolism.

Sources of vitamin B6 include bananas, tuna, chicken breast, roasted turkey, and salmon.Vitamin B6 deficiency symptomsThe symptoms of pyridoxine deficiencies are fatigue, anemia, convulsion, and eczema.[xvi]

7. Vitamin B7 or biotin or vitamin H Biotin breaks down fatty acids and carbohydrates in order to produce energy, it promotes the synthesis of proteins in order to build up muscles. It also promotes nervous-system activities (sensation and motion). Sources of biotin include swiss chard.

Biotin deficiency causes *cradle cap* in children, seborrheic dermatitis in adult, hair loss, seizure, muscle cramps, lack of muscle coordination, hypotonia, inability of efficient sugar use in the body for energy production.

8. Folic acid or vitamin B9 plays an important role in blood-cell synthesis: it prevents *spina bifida*. Deficiency in folic acid causes *anemia.* Anemia is a condition in which there is a deficit in healthy or normal red blood cells, which carry oxygen to body cells.

Sources of folic acid

Lentils, sunflowers, orange juice, grapes, pineapples, asparagus, spinach, and okra.

9. Vitamin B12 (Cyanocobalamine) is useful for DNA synthesis, proper red blood cells' synthesis, and neurological function.

Sources of vitamin B12

Meat, milk, liver, fish, poultry, eggs, and nutritional-yeast products.

Vitamin B12 deficiency causes *megaloblastic anemia,* which is a condition characterized by larger red blood cells.

10. Vitamin C, or ascorbic acid, is the most abundant water-soluble antioxidant in a human body. It boosts the immune system and prevents many diseases: for example, gout and Respiratory Tract Infections. It can also do the following:

• Promote the repairing of body cells

• Have antiaging properties

• Protect the skin

• Burn up fat

• Maintain healthy bone mass

• Maintain a healthy heart and eyes

• Promote iron absorption

• Decrease the risk of developing cancer, especially of the mouth, laryngeal, and esophageal types

• Restore vitamin E to its active form

Sources of vitamin C

Oranges, lemons, and mandarins all contain vitamin C.

NB: Increased intake of omega 3 vitamin E and C decreases the risk of developing pancreatic cancer.[xvii]

Vitamin C and E repair traumatic brain injury.

Vitamin C deficiency may impair brain development and it may cause asthma. In children the lack of vitamin C may cause mental and memory troubles.

Lack of vitamin C may cause scurvy.

Scurvy is a condition characterized by anemia, weakness, bleeding gums, muscular and cutaneous hemorrhage.

11. Vitamin D promotes calcium absorption, regulates the level of calcium and phosphate in your body, and regulates normal mineralization of bones. Vitamin D is also necessary for bone growth and bone remodeling (the process of reshaping).

Vitamin D promotes cell growth and neuromuscular and immunologic function; it decreases inflammation.

Sources of vitamin D

Vitamin D is present in very few foods: flesh of fatty fish such as salmon and tuna, fish's liver, beef liver, cheese, egg yolk, and mushrooms.

Vitamin D is also produced inside the body when the sun's rays touch the body cholesterol found under the skin.

Deficiency in vitamin D is characterized by the following:

• Ossification disorders; nodular enlargement on the ends and sides of bones

• Delay of fontanel's closure

• Muscle pains and sweating

• Distortion of bones and bonding bones

• Rickets in children

- Osteomalacia in adults

- Osteoporosis in old age

12. Vitamin E is powerful and the most abundant fat-soluble antioxidant in the body; it protects cells from damaging effects caused by free radicals, prevents LDL oxidation and the formation of clogging plaques in arteries.

Sources of vitamin E

Nuts, seeds, vegetable oil, fortified seeds, leafy vegetables

13. Vitamin K deficiency causes coagulation disorders.

Sources of vitamin K

Green vegetables, mustard seeds, broccoli, cauliflowers, kale, lettuces, cabbage, spinach, carrots, avocado, green peas, apples, asparagus, grapes, beef, chicken, fish, turkey, canola oil, olive oil, and mayonnaise.

14. Calcium is the most abundant mineral in a human being's body. Calcium is very important for healthy bones and strong teeth. Calcium regulates heart rhythm and blood pressure, and it plays an important role in muscle contraction and relaxation; it also regulates hormonal and nerve function.

Sources of calcium

Dairy products; seafood; dried beans; nuts; cereals; green, leafy vegetables; and bread.

There are two kinds of calcium deficiencies:

1. *Osteoporosis*: Condition characterized by tiny and weak bones and caused by an inadequate intake of calcium.

2. *Hypocalcaemia*: Low calcium level in the blood caused by some diseases—for example, kidney failure, hypoparathyroidism, or by the intake of some medicines (e.g., diuretics).

NB: Inadequate supply of dietary calcium may not lead to *hypocalcaemia*, but it will lead to osteoporosis, because your system will take calcium from your bones to respond to its physiologic needs.

15. Potassium: It is a mineral that maintains water and acid balance (PH) in the blood and cell tissues. It regulates the transmission of the body's electric signals between nerves and body cells; it regulates a good function of cells, tissues, and organs. It regulates muscle-building.

Sources of Potassium

Bananas, orange juice, avocado, cantaloupes, tomatoes, potatoes, lima beans, salmon, and meats

Potassium deficiency or *hypocaliemia* causes dry skin, dizziness, fatigue, irritability, anxiety, restlessness, confusion, depression, slow reflexes, muscle cramps, spasm, hypertension, heart dysrythmia, chest pains, paralysis, osteoporosis, and kidney failure.

NB: Hypocaliemia is a medical emergency, as it may easily stop the heart.

Causes of potassium deficiency

• Diet poor in potassium: this usually happens when an individual is eating food rich in sodium chloride.

• Diseases that cause anorexia, and or excessive vomiting and diarrhea, in such a way that a person is not able to absorb potassium.

Excessive sweating, hyperthyroidism, anemia, crushing disease, kidney disease, uncontrollable diabetes mellitus

• Some medicines (e.g., diuretics, cortisone).

16. Magnesium is a very important mineral for the biochemical reactions in the human body. It promotes good health, regulates nerves and muscle function, supports the immune system, regulates the cardiac rhythm, promotes normal blood pressure, controls blood sugar, and maintains strong and healthy bones. Magnesium is involved in protein synthesis and energy production.

About fifty percent of magnesium is found in bones, another approximately fifty percent of it in body cells, and only one percent is found in blood.

Sources of magnesium

Green vegetables	Nuts
Beans	Seeds
Peas	Whole grains

Magnesium deficiency causes excessive electrical activity in the brain, which may lead to the change of behavior, numbness, tingling, muscle contraction, cramps, and seizure.

Causes of magnesium deficiency

• Gastrointestinal disorders such as vomiting, diarrhea and Crohn's disease, kidney disease, uncontrollable diabetes mellitus, alcohol abuse

• Some medicines such as diuretics, antibiotic *(gentamycin)*, *antineoplastic medications (cisplatin)*, *hypocalcemia, hypocaliemia*

17. Iron is an important mineral in a human body and plays a major role in synthesizing red blood cells.

Sources of iron

Red meat, liver, turkey and chicken giblets, dairy products, egg yolks, dark green leafy vegetables, avocado, dried fruits (raisins), beans, lentils, soybeans, iron enriched cereals and grains, mollusks, and artichokes.

deficiency of iron causes *anemia.* Causes of iron deficiency include the following:

Lack of iron in diet

Pregnancy

Hemorrhages
Diseases such as malaria

OBESITY

"Obesity is defined as an excessive accumulation of fats in the body."[xviii]

Causes of obesity

Heredity

Lack of activity (that is associated with good appetite)

Wrong choice of nutrients: per example when an individual is eating sugary rich food and too much fat.

NB: Depression and stress increase appetite.

Treatment

• Diet: Decrease your intake of fats, carbohydrates, and proteins, but eat more high-fiber foods, as they fill you up without loading you up with calories.

• Exercise

• Deal with stress

HIGH CHOLESTEROL

For you to understand having high *cholesterol*, you have first to know what *cholesterol* is. *Cholesterol* is a waxy, insoluble substance produced by the liver. It may also be supplied to an individual through ingestion of some specific foods, especially animal products.

Cholesterol forms an important part of cell membranes; it is useful for the ability of different organs of our bodies to work. *Cholesterol* in association with the sun's rays produces vitamin D.

Cholesterol allows the synthesis of bile acid; this is useful for the absorption of fat by body tissues.

Cholesterol is also useful for the absorption of hormones (e.g., testosterone, estrogens, progesterone, and cortisol).

High cholesterol is defined as the presence of an abnormally large amount of *cholesterol* in the blood.[xix]

Lipoproteins enable the transport of cholesterol into the bloodstream. There are two different kinds of *lipoproteins:* LDL and HDL.

LDL (low-density lipoprotein), OR BAD CHOLESTEROL

LDL transports cholesterol from the liver to the body tissues, where it may be used, but the human body does not need a large amount of it.

The excessive amount of LDL promotes accumulation of *cholesterol* in the bloodstream. This can cause a total blockage of a vessel and lead to a heart attack when it is accumulated in the heart vessel (coronary arteries).

It can also lead to a stroke, depending on the area of the affected brain vessel.

These are the reasons why *low density lipoprotein* is commonly called bad cholesterol.

NB: LDL oxidation in association with a high level of sugar in the bloodstream may damage *endothelium* (the cells lining arteries).[xx]

Roles of endothelium

• It regulates blood pressure by promoting dilatation or constriction of blood vessels.

• It regulates blood clotting.

• It regulates the volume of fluids and the level of electrolytes.

• It regulates the passage of nutrients, hormones, and medicines from the bloodstream to the body tissues.

• It regulates the body's immune response to germs.

All of these functions may be possible only if the endothelium is not damaged.

NB: Damaged *endothelium* causes cholesterol plaques to form in the arteries.

LDL is found in the following foods

• Tripe and casings

• Wurst and sausages

• Cheese

• All birds' fat tissues, skins, and feet

• All animal's fat tissues, skins, and legs

What to do about the excessive amount of LDL or bad cholesterol?

• Avoid eating big amounts of food rich in LDL or bad *cholesterol*.

• Eat enough food rich in HDL or good *cholesterol*.

Olive oil decreases LDL and increases HDL; it is also very rich in antioxidants.

Red wine (taken moderately) increases HDL but does not decrease LDL. An average of one glass of red wine a day is reasonable.

Foods rich in soluble fibers such as apples, pears, prunes, grains, oatmeals, and beans lower LDL and raise HDL.

Exercise to burn up and eliminate the bad cholesterol.

HDL (High-density lipoprotein) OR GOOD CHOLESTEROL

HDL takes back cholesterol to the liver. It inhibits oxidation of LDL and prevents accumulation of cholesterol in the bloodstream. It removes cholesterol from the vessel's walls. HDL also prevents blood from clotting in the vessels.

That is why it is called good *cholesterol*. [xxi]

Sources of HDL

• Fish, such as salmon, tuna, halibut, and mackerel

- Nuts, such as almond, walnuts, and cashews

4. EXERCISE

Exercise is a physical activity done on a regular basis with the purpose of becoming healthier or stronger.

ADVANTAGES OF EXERCISE

Exercise is very good and very important for people of all ages:

• It helps you to release *catecholamine* (hormone produced by your body while having stress and which is responsible for high blood pressure).

• It strengthens cardiac muscles and reduces the risk of cardiac disease.

• It decreases the LDL.

• It increases HDL.

• It decreases the fat around the body.

• It helps to control the level of blood sugar.

• It strengthens bones.

- It gives muscle strength.

- It improves your immune system.

- It gives energy.

- It releases stress.

5. PROBLEMS ACCORDING TO

AGE

In this chapter you will find diseases according to age groups, but those diseases may also be found in people of all ages. (I did specify that the disease is either frequent or more serious to a specific age group.)

CHILDHOOD

PSYCHOLOGICAL PROBLEMS

SOME PSYCHOLOGICAL NEEDS FOR CHILDREN

All children need to be loved, especially by their parents. Parents' love stimulates the child's mental and physical development. Love helps children develop self-confidence. When a child does not feel loved, he may not perform well at school and may even suffer from depression.

Children like parental attention. When a parent or guardian does not take interest in the child, she may misbehave seeking for attention.

Children like to feel accepted by their parents and to belong to a family. This makes them feel secure.

All children need to be respected. The lack of respect may lead to lack of self-esteem.

All children need guidance to achieve success.

All children need protection from all kinds of danger. This will help them to feel safe.

All children need to be encouraged and congratulated for the good things they do. Let them know that they have done well or carried out an instruction. Always remember to thank the child for a job well done.

All children need friendship; encourage them to socialize.

All children need to feel that they may make their own choices sometimes. Encourage them to make good choices.

All children need their parents to provide for their needs.

SOME OF THE PSYCHOLOGICAL PROBLEMS CHILDREN MAY FACE

Children may face developmental, emotional, behavioral, and social problems such as fearfulness, anxiety, aggressiveness, attachment disorder, being overstressed, depression, misconduct, social withdrawal, impulsivity, and low self-esteem.

CAUSES OF PSYCHOLOGICAL PROBLEMS IN CHILDREN

Some of the causes of psychological problems in children are their parents' divorce, losing a parent or guardian, domestic violence, car accidents, the diagnosis of a chronic disease, hospitalization, witnessing a bad event (e.g., when a child witnesses robbers torturing an individual), and physical and sexual abuse.

NB: Please consult your nearest clinic or your child's doctor for advice, once you notice any of these problems in your child.

MALNUTRITION

UNDERNOURISHMENT

A child may develop malnutrition (undernourishment) if he or she is not well fed. To prevent a child from being malnourished, a suitable and balanced diet is important. To feed a child involves a choice of nutrients that are suitable for the body's growth and given or prepared in a way that the body can assimilate them easily.

Malnutrition or undernourishment affects the physical and mental growth of children.

Children who suffer from undernourishment may not perform well at school. This situation may lead to problems as the child gets older.

OBESITY

Children can also develop obesity if they are overfed and do not exercise.

Today's children do not play much outside, and they watch television for long hours or play electronic games, which do not help them to let loose energy and burn calories, and as a consequence, they become obese.

Children must be encouraged to play soccer, ride a bicycle, swim, skip a rope, and to run and to jump, so they can burn up fat and avoid obesity.

PHYSICAL PROBLEMS

INFLUENZA

Influenza, or flu, is a disease caused by viruses called *influenza*. There are three kinds of *influenza* viruses: A, B, and C. These viruses are found in the air and can affect the respiratory system of human beings, animals, and birds. This disease is very contagious, and the contamination is made via the nose while breathing. Viruses may also spread when an individual touches anything that is infected by the flu virus and then touches his or her own eyes, nose, or mouth. An infected person starts to spread the disease one day before the evidence of symptoms and up to seven days later. Children may spread the disease for a little longer.

An infected person releases viruses while sneezing, coughing, laughing, talking, and breathing. *Influenza* viruses may survive outside the body up to eight hours, but this virus is sensitive to heat, soap, and chemicals. *Influenza* is a common disease, especially during winter.[xxii]

Symptoms

• Sneezing

• Coughing

• Running nose

• Headache

• Fever

Some individuals, especially children, may present more symptoms, which are sore throat, nausea, vomiting, and diarrhea.

Prevention

• Avoid sitting next to someone suffering from flu, or make sure the distance between you and that person is at least 50 cm.

• Wash your hands with soap after you have touched an infected person, or after you have touched whatever that person had been using.

• Teach children to use tissue to cover their mouths while coughing or sneezing and to throw the tissue away in the trash can, and to use sanitizers (if it is allowed by the manufacture and if it is safe, or otherwise to wash hands) before they touch anything (this measure will help prevent them from spreading the disease).

• Protect or cover yourself very well, especially your neck, chest, and feet.

• Drink hot tea regularly, to warm up yourself.

• Eat enough vegetables and fruits, especially lemons and oranges, to boost your immune system.

• Exercise regularly to boost your immune system.

• Consult your clinic for a flu vaccine.

What must I do when I notice the symptoms of flu?

• Rest.

• Cover your body properly, especially your neck.

• Take enough nutrients rich in vitamin C.

• Drink hot tea.

• Take painkillers.

• Consult your nearest clinic or doctor as soon as possible to make sure that it is a simple flu and not pneumonia.

Complications of flu

To people with immune depression (pregnant women, cancer patients, diabetic, and people affected by AIDS, arthritis, and depression), a simple flu can complicate with a viral pneumonia; it can also make you vulnerable to a bacterial pneumonia. Flu can kill

Beware

When your heater is on, open your windows slightly to allow passage of oxygen in the room. Never sleep with a heater on. Beware of the danger of gas heater, especially when you have children.

Make sure there is no one suffering from TB among the people in the room. (If a person has been on TB treatment for more than two weeks, he can not transmit the disease anymore, but he must continue and complete his treatment; otherwise, he cannot be healed unless he complete his treatment.)

Avoid very hot and full water bottles. Close your hot water bottles after releasing the air to avoid pressure that could otherwise break them.

Beware of children when you are making tea.

Never forget that you still need oxygen in the house, even when it is very cold. You can sit in a bedroom for ten minutes and open all the windows in the living room to allow the fresh air to penetrate into the living room, especially if there are many people in the house. This can be done several times a day.

ASTHMA

"Asthma is not an infectious disease, but it is a chronic inflammatory disorder with reversible airway obstruction. In susceptible patients, exposure to various environmental triggers, allergens, or viral infections stimuli results in inflammatory changes, bronchospasm, increased bronchial secretions, mucus plugs formation, and, if not controlled, eventual bronchial muscle hypertrophy of the airway's smooth muscle. All these factors contribute to airway obstruction."[xxiii]

Causes

• Genetic predisposition in association with environmental lifestyle factors, such as those listed below.

Risk factors of asthma in a child

Asthma history in the family.

Prematurity and low weight at birth.

Presence of an allergen.

Frequent respiratory-tract infections.

Secondhand smoking.

Sex: males are more likely to develop asthma than are females.

Children who are not breast-fed may develop asthma more easily than others, because they lack the antibody from breast milk.

Symptoms

Asthma symptoms are different from one child to another, and, even for the same child, symptoms differ from one episode to another.

Common symptoms are as follows:

Coughing and wheezing chest—but not all coughs or wheezing are caused by asthma.

Short and rapid breath.

Loss of energy while playing.

Chest pain.

Frequent headaches.

NB: Asthma may start at any age, but its diagnosis is not easy, especially in children under the age of two years. It is only after two years of age that the diagnosis of asthma may be made.

Treatment

Prevention

• Stop secondhand smoking.

• Avoid dust.

• Avoid exposure to identified allergens.

• Avoid contact with pets.

Medical treatment

Consult a clinic or your child's doctor as soon as you notice the first symptom of asthma or any respiratory-tract disease in your child.

Asthma being a chronic condition, an asthmatic patient must always carry inhalers (corticoid/bronchodilators).[xxiv]

TONSILLITIS

For you to understand this chapter, you have first to know what tonsils are. You have two kinds of tonsils: palatine and nasopharyngeal.

Palatine tonsils: Lymphoid tissues situated at the posterior and lateral part of the throat, one at the left and another at the right side. Their role is to produce specific antibodies to fight against inhaled or ingested germs.

Nasopharyngeal tonsils or *adenoids*: Lymphoid tissues situated in the posterior part of the nose in the upper and anterior part of the throat. Adenoids may be inflamed and affect breathing and speech.

Tonsillitis is an inflammation of one or both tonsils caused by a viral or bacterial infection. A viral tonsillitis may be complicated by a bacterial one.

In most cases group A beta hemolytic streptococci (germ) is responsible for the disease.

Tonsillitis is contagious: it spreads when a sick patient is coughing, sneezing, talking, or laughing. It can also be spread by kissing or sharing a cup or spoon with an infected person.

Risk factors of tonsillitis

• Young age: children are more vulnerable than adults.

• Frequent exposure to germs.

• Secondhand smoking.

Symptoms

• Sore throat

• Difficulty in swallowing

- Fever (a body temperature may reach 40∘C)

- Malaises

- Headache

- Nausea and vomiting

Complications

- Chronic tonsillitis

- Rhinitis (inflammation of the nasal mucous membranes)

- Peritonsillar abscess

- Deep neck abscess

- Cervical lymph-nodes abscess

- Sinusitis

- Otitis media

- Rheumatic fever

• Glomerulonephritis (inflammatory disease of the kidney)

• Pneumonia (lungs infection)

• Osteomyelitis (inflammation of the bone marrow)

• Infectious endocarditis (inflammation of the internal layer of the heart)

Prevention

• Protect your child from being exposed to germs by avoiding contact with an infected person.

• Teach your child to wash hands or to use sanitizers regularly.

• Clean and disinfect your house properly and your child's toys.

• Teach your child to cover the mouth, using a tissue, while coughing or sneezing.

• Protect your child from secondhand smoking.

Treatment

• Bed rest.

• Fluid intake.

• Light diet.

• Consult a doctor for medical treatment (antibiotics and painkillers).

NB: A child must complete his antibiotic course.

A removal of tonsils may be a solution in some cases.[xxv]

SINUSITIS

For you to understand what sinusitis is, you must know first what a sinus is. A sinus is a cavity within a bone, mostly found in face bones connected with the nasal cavity.

Sinusitis is an infection of sinuses that mostly occurs after an upper respiratory-tract infection, tonsillitis, or an upper dental abscess or extraction.

Symptoms

• Pain, tenderness, redness, and swelling at the area of the affected sinus

• Blocked nose

• Purulent nasal discharge

• Infection's signs (fever, malaises, headache)

NB: The headache is severe during the day.

Complications

• Chronic sinusitis

• Facial abscess

• Osteomyelitis (inflammation of bones marrow) of facial bones

• Meningitis (Inflammation of layers that cover the brain)

• Brain abscess

Prevention

Protect your children from colds and flu; if they are affected, make sure that they receive proper care.

Assure good dental and mouth hygiene for your children, and get them treated as soon as you notice any abnormality in their mouths.

Make sure that you child has proper care after a dental extraction.

Treatment

• Bed rest.

• Consult a doctor for medical treatment (antibiotics and pain killers).

• Drainage may be needed in serious cases.

NB: A child must complete his antibiotic course.[xxvi]

ACUTE OTITIS MEDIA

Otitis media is an infection of the middle part of the ear. Acute otitis is a common disease in children, because their Eustachian tubes are narrow and horizontal, allowing the passage of germs from the throat to the ear. Most of the time, the disease appears after an upper respiratory-tract infection, sinusitis, or tonsillitis.

The infection causes the inflammation of the ear lining; white blood cells accumulate themselves to fight the infection and end up dying, converting themselves into pus.

Germs found in most cases of otitis:

• *Haemophilus influenzoe*

• *Streptococcus pneumoniae*

• *Maraxela catarrhalis*

Otitis risk factors

• Secondhand smoking

•Allergies

•Congenital malformation of the palate (e.g., in a case of cleft palate)

• Nursing a child from a bottle while lying down.

• Maltreated upper-respiratory infection.

Symptoms

• Ear pain

• Discharging ear

• Blocked ear

• Fever

• Malaises

• Vomiting

Complications

- Chronic otitis

- Perforation of eardrum

- Necrosis of eardrum

- Hearing loss

- Mastoiditis (inflammation of a part of a bone found behind the ear)

- Facial nerve paralysis

- Meningitis (Infection of layers that cover the brain)

NB: Otitis media, to a child, is a medical emergency.

Treatment

- Bed rest.

- Consult a doctor for medical treatment (antibiotics and painkillers).

• In some cases ear drainage or a therapeutic incision of the tympanic membrane may be needed.

NB: A child must complete his antibiotic course.[xxvii]

EPILEPSY

Epilepsy is not an infectious disease but the most frequent neurological disorder affecting all ages and characterized by a recurrent seizure. Epilepsy being a chronic disease, the treatment is for life.

NB: Epilepsy may not be curable, but in seventy percent of cases it may be very well managed.

Causes

• Lack of oxygen during birth process; this can happen when labor is delayed.

(NB: The lack of oxygen will provoke cerebral ischemia, which leads to encephalopathy.)

• Central nervous system infection.

• Central nervous system abnormality.

• Central nervous system lesion (head trauma affecting the brain).

• Brain tumors.

• Metabolic disorders.

To an adult, other causes of epilepsy are stress, alcohol withdrawal, and drug abuse.

What to do when a child has a fit

• Roll the child on his side to prevent inhalation of fluids from the stomach (regurgitation).

• Open belt, clothes zippers and buttons.

• Remove the child's shoes.

• Make sure there are no hazards around the child. Per example a stone, a knife, a kettle filled in with hot water

• Aerate the room.

• Record the date, time, and duration of seizure in a special book.

• Call an ambulance if the fit takes more than five minutes.

NB: In some cases a neurosurgery may be a solution to decrease the frequency of fits or to cure, according to the case.[xxviii]

REPRODUCTIVE PERIOD

During the reproductive period a person can face problems that are discussed in the following sections.

PSYCHOLOGICAL PROBLEMS

During puberty, sexual glands start to produce hormones, which affect character and body. The young person does not understand what is going on, becomes irritable and restless, and has an impression that no one understands him, because he does not understand himself either. This can lead to depression.

Teenagers need to be loved, they need assurance and understanding, and they need encouragement when they do good; they need to be valued and to be guided in the right way. They need an available adult to whom they can express themselves, who can explain to them what is going on, and who can correct them without harm but with love.

Abuse: Misuse or wrong use, particularly excessive use, of anything. Abuse can be emotional, physical, or sexual. Abuse can be a one-time or a continuous experience and may lead to depression. In most cases, lack of confidence is a consequence of emotional abuse.

NB: If you find yourself in any of these situations, you need to quickly consult your nearest clinic or your family doctor for referral if necessary.[xxix]

DEPRESSION

"Depression is defined in the dictionary as a hollow or depressed area; downward or inward displacement; a lowering or decreasing of functional activity.

Depression is also a psychiatric syndrome consisting of dejected mood, psychomotor retardation, insomnia, and weight loss, sometimes associated with guilt feelings and somatic preoccupations, often of delusional proportions."[xxx]

Causes

• Gender: Females are much more vulnerable to depression than males.

• Heredity (when someone in your family is suffering from Depression you are at risk of developing it): per example when you mother is suffering from Depression.

• Socioeconomic situations: per example when you loses your job.

• Affective problems: per example when you find out that your partner is cheating on you.

• Abuse: per example when a person is always wrongly accused.

• Lack of self-confidence is a consequence of emotional abuse and once you loses your self confidence you becomes a subject to all kind of abuses.

Symptoms

• Fluctuation of mood, swinging from sadness to hopelessness.

• Inability to concentrate and lack of decisiveness.

• Loss of interest.

• Presence of some physical symptoms such as headache, running stomach, constipation, insomnia, anorexia, or bulimia.

• Anxiety

- Psychomotor retardation

- Persecutory nature

- Withdrawal from activities

- Suicidal thoughts

How do I prevent depression?

Consult the nearest clinic or your family doctor as soon as you notice the first symptoms and/or you find yourself within a situation that may lead to depression.

Treatment

Consult your nearest clinic or your family doctor for assessment and referral.

PHYSICAL PROBLEMS

Some symptoms women may present during the reproductive period:

• Difficult and painful menstruations

• Excessively prolonged or diffuse menses

• Abnormally frequent menses

• Little quantity or absence of menses

• Absence or abnormal cessation of menses

• Sterility—the fact of being unable to conceive while having normal and frequent unprotected sexual intercourse

• "Miscarriage—spontaneous expulsion of the product of pregnancy before the middle of the second trimester"[xxxi]

• "Premature labor—onset of labor before the thirty-seventh completed week of pregnancy dated from the last normal menstruation period"[xxxii]

- Lower abdomen pains

- Lower back pains

- Spinal cord pains

- Bad smelling vaginal discharge

- Burning urine

- Itching vagina

- Presence of an ulcer or lump on the vulva

- Lump on breast

- Bleeding breast

- Painful breast

- Flow of milk from the breast other than normal lactation

When any of these symptoms is present, a woman must consult the nearest clinic or doctor for investigation.

Boys may experience a suddenly painful testis (this is an extreme surgical emergency).

SEXUALLY TRANSMISSIBLE DISEASE (STD)

An STD is a disease that an individual gets by having unprotected sexual intercourse with an infected person, by sharing towels or panties with an infected person, or by sharing a non-disinfected toilet with an infected person.

Symptoms

• Itching vagina/ Burning or pain in passing urine (penis pain)

• Lower abdomen pains

• Lower back pains

• Excessive vaginal discharges

• Change in vaginal discharge color and odor

• Urethral discharge (men)

NB: Men present symptoms of STD earlier, because of the length of their urethra and their urine using the same affected urethra.

Women present symptoms of STD very late, because they do not use the vagina to pass urine. The urine does not touch the affected area, which is the vagina. As a consequence a woman can be passing infections to people without her knowing.

Does STD cure totally?

Yes, but there are conditions:

• The patient must take the medication correctly and complete the course.

• All partners must be treated properly, even when they do not present any symptoms.

• Avoid unprotected sex while still taking medication.

Complications of STD

If a specific STD is not treated at its early stage, as many of STDs do not present symptoms early, the following complications may occur:

- Body bumps

- Recurrent genital sores

- Generalized skin rash

- Groin abscess

- Eye inflammation

- Arthritis

- Infertility

- Cervical cancer

VULVO- VAGINAL IRRITATION

Vulvo-vaginal irritation is a condition characterized by the presence of rash, burning, and soreness of both vagina and vulva.

Causes

1. Natural: the moisture of the vulva's skin (after passing urine or during menstruation) together with frequent frictions while moving makes it extremely sensitive and vulnerable.

2. Allergy: some women react to hygienic products made with plastic, cellulose, or viscose.

3. Chemicals: in the vagina we find saprophyte bacteria that produce acid to neutralize *Candida albicans*.

Using soap on these private parts may kill those bacteria that condition would otherwise promote the emergence of fungal infection and cause irritation.

Chemicals found in new panties, pads, tampons, panty liners, toilet tissues, new towels, or laundry soap and detergent (used to wash or disinfect panties) can also cause burning and irritations.

4. Infections: using petro-chemical products on the genitals can create a suitable environment for the proliferation of germs and cause infection and irritation.

5. Trauma: in a case of a traumatic intercourse or rape.

6. Other irritants

- Wet panties

- Infected panties

- Strings

- Tight clothing or underwear

2. How to prevent the vulvo-vaginal irritation.

To prevent vulvo-vaginal irritation, you have to do the following:

1. Use 100-percent-cotton hygienic products.

2. Avoid wearing wet panties; if possible expose them to the sun, as the sun's rays kill most germs.

3. Wash the vulva at least once a day with water but without soap, as soap may change the natural pH of the vagina.

4. Wipe yourself properly after you have used the toilet: a woman must wipe herself from the front to the back and not vice versa, as wiping from the back to the front can bring germs from the anus to the vulva and cause infection and irritation.

NB: Some germs can be harmless to the digestive tract but harmful somewhere else.

5. Wash new panties and new towels before usage.

6. Rinse panties and towels properly.[xxxiii]

VAGINAL CANDIDIASIS OR YEAST INFECTION

Vaginal candidiasis is the infection caused by *Candida albicans* (a fungus). This is not an STD.

All human beings have some *Candida albicans* in their digestive tracts, skin, and, for women, their vaginas. These fungi are harmless to healthy individuals, as healthy people have strong immune systems. Immune depression promotes the emergence of candidiasis.

Causes of immune depression

1. Natural—e.g., in a case of pregnancy

2. Diseases—e.g., in a case of AIDS, diabetes mellitus (sugar diabetic), rheumatoid arthritis, or cancer

3. Medicines—e.g., from steroids, some oral contraceptives with high estrogen content, or cancer chemotherapy.

4. Stress and depression may also weaken the immune system and contribute to the emergence of the disease.

5. Local irritation and allergic reaction may also weaken the immune system and contribute to the emergence of vaginal candidiasis.

Apart from in the immune system, in the vagina we find saprophytes bacteria, which produce acid to neutralize vaginal candida.

Some antibiotics taken for a long period may kill those bacteria and contribute to the emergence of candidiasis.

The use of some chemicals such as soap to the genitals may also kill those saprophytes bacteria and contribute to the emergence of the disease.

Vaginal douching changes the vaginal pH, which becomes alkaline and promotes local inflammation, which in turn contributes to the emergence of the disease.

Symptoms

• Smelly, thick, white yellowish discharge

•Itching, burning, and painful urination

• Painful intercourse

• Difficulty on walking because of the pain

Prevention

• Avoid vaginal douching, because it changes the vaginal pH and causes inflammation, which may increase the risk of the disease.

• While washing your panties, avoid using powder soap, fabric softeners, or bleach, which may harm vaginal bacteria that produce acid that neutralize candida.

• Wear cotton underwear.

• Avoid washing the vagina/vulva with soap or bubble-bath products.

Diet and treatment

• Reduce or avoid sugar, as it allows candida to grow very fast and to become harmful.

• Avoid alcohol, as it converts into sugar.

• Eat enough garlic, especially when it's fresh.

• Drink milk or eat yogurts rich in acidophilus bacteria.

• Consult your nearest clinic or doctor for medical treatment.[xxxiv]

CANCER

Cancer is an abnormal tissue that grow rapidly and continuously by cellular replication

BREAST CANCER

Cause

Like other cancers, there is no proper or clear and direct cause of breast cancer, but there are risk factors:

• *Heredity.*

• *Women with three or more children have a lower incidence than women with few children.*

• *Every pregnancy before the age of thirty appears to reduce the risk of breast cancer.*

• *Menarche (first menstruation) after fifteen years of age and artificial menopause is also associated with a lower incidence of breast cancer, whereas early menarche (under twelve years old) and late natural menopause (after fifty years) is associated with a slight increase in the risk of developing breast cancer.*

• *Presence of breast cyst.*

• *Cancer in opposite breast—a woman who has cancer in one breast is at increased risk of developing cancer in the opposite breast.*

• *Cancer of uterus and ovary—women with cancer of uterus corpus have a risk of getting breast cancer, almost double that of the general population.*

• *Breast trauma.*

• *Oral contraceptives and menopausal estrogens."*[xxxv]

• Abortion.

Symptoms

Stage 1: Usually there is no pain at the beginning of the process. The mass is hard and irregular, with nipple erosion.

Stage 2: At this stage there is retraction of the nipple, redness of the axillary lymph nodes, pain and enlargement of the breast, edema, and fixation of the mass to the skin or chest.

Stage 3: This is the last stage, where you find ulceration, supra clavicular lymph node(s), arm edema, and metastases.

NB: Mammography can detect breast cancer at its early stage.

Breast examination

Every woman needs to be able to examine her own breasts. There are normal variations in breast tissues during the menstruation cycle, pregnancy, and during menopause. This must be distinguished from the pathologic variations. Many women complain of tenderness and lumpiness before their menstruation periods; that is the reason why it is recommended that women should proceed on breast examination only after the menses: from the fifth day of the cycle. Breasts should be examined standing and lying down.

The best place to examine your breasts is in front of a large mirror. To facilitate the manipulation, a woman can rub her breasts with a body lotion or cream. She can also use any foam solution.

How to examine breasts

Step 1: Stand before a large mirror. Look at both breasts carefully and check if there is any abnormality in size, color, or shape.

Step 2: Clasp your hands behind your head.

Press your elbows forward. Check the contour of your breasts. Compare breasts to each other and look for any change.

Step 3: Put your hands firmly on your hip.

Bow slightly toward your mirror as you pull forward your elbows and check very well the contour of your breasts.

Step 4: Put your left hand behind your head.

Use the flat surface of your right hand to palpate firmly and carefully your left breast.

Start with the outer edge of your breast: do a small circle with the flat surface of your fingers, move slowly in a circle around your breast, and move gradually towards your nipple, making sure that you palpate the whole breast.

Check carefully the space between your breasts and the armpit. Check for any lump or mass under the skin.

Press the nipple, and check to find out if there is any discharge.

Keep the hand flat at the breast.

Repeat the process on your right breast.

Step 5: Lie flat on your back. Put a pillow under your left shoulder. Put your left arm under your head. Restart step 4.

What is the prognosis in a case of breast cancer?

The prognosis depends on the stage at which the diagnosis is made. The earlier the diagnosis is made, the more an accurate prognosis is made possible.

"Cancer of the cervix is the third most-common malignancy in women (exceeded only by breast and colon cancer)".[xxxvi]

Symptoms

In the early stage of cervical cancer, it is not easy to distinguish between symptoms of cervical cancer and those of other pelvic affections. In many cases women take those symptoms for premenstrual pain or ovulation pain.

At a later stage, symptoms become more serious in the case of cervical cancer, but this is different from one woman to another.

Common symptoms

• Abnormal bleeding vagina.

• Unusually heavy vaginal discharge.

• Bleeding between regular menstruation periods, after pelvic examination, and after sex.

• Severe lower abdominal pain.

Painful urine (this happens when the cancer has already spread to the urinary system).

Causes and prevention

"The cause of cervical cancer is still unknown. Nevertheless, complete chastity is associated with almost total freedom from this malignancy. Theoretically, carcinoma of the cervix before middle age may be considered to be a carcinogen-induced neoplasm. The incidence of cervical cancer should therefore be reduced by the following measures:

• Improved personal hygiene

• Prevention and prompt treatment of vaginitis (infection of the vagina) and cervicitis (infection of the uterine cervix)

• Avoidance of sexual intercourse at an early age

• Limitation of the number of sexual partners

• *Frequent cancer cytoscreening of all women, especially parous individuals in deprived social circumstances and those who have had many sexual partners*

• *Prompt removal of suspect cervical lesions, such as epithelial anaplasia, dysplasia, and atypical or equivocal foci"*[xxxvii]

Prognosis

The earlier the diagnosis is made, the better prognosis for proper treatment.

PEPTIC ULCER DISEASE

Peptic ulcer is an excavation that develops in the esophagus, gastric, or duodenal (first part of the small intestine) mucosa.

Symptoms

• Upper abdomen discomfort or pain

• Tenderness of the upper abdomen

• Heartburn

• Sensation of full stomach

• Nausea, vomiting, and loss of appetite

• Hemorrhage may be present; in such a case, a patient will vomit up blood (hematemesis) or may release black stools (melena).

Causes

In most cases the cause is unknown, but in some cases causes are as listed below:

• Infection: a bacteria called *Helicobacter pylori* can cause peptic ulcer disease.

• Hyperacidity: When a person undergoes a stressful situation, his gastric glands produce more acids, as if she was digesting food in her stomach. This will make the gastric mucosa digested by gastric acid, and she will develop an ulcer.

• An endocrine tumor–producing acid

• Benign and malignant tumor of the pancreas, secreting gastrin

• Tobacco inhibits the secretion of bicarbonate by the pancreas; this condition raises the acidity level in the duodenum and contributes to the emergence of ulcer.

•Chemical: some medicines inhibit the secretion of the mucus that protects gastric mucosa from gastric acid damage. Among them we do find reserpine and NSAIDs (nonsteroidal anti-inflammatory drugs) .

Some NSAIDs are *salicylates, indomethacin, diclofenac, ibuprofen.*

Alcohol.

Predisposition factors

• Familial tendency

• Chronic pulmonary infection

• Chronic renal infection

Treatment

Diet

• Stop consuming alcohol and smoking.

• Stop irritants such as lemon, vinegar, chili, atchaar, chakalaka, tomato sauce, spices, coke, coffee, or sour milk.

• Take three regular meals daily (for as long as you are still taking your medicines) or take small regular meals, but avoid eating in between.

• Avoid very hot or very cold meals.

• Drink enough lukewarm water but little by little.

Medical treatment

Consult your family doctor for assessment and medical treatment (antibiotics, histamine II receptor antagonist /antacids)

• Antibiotic kills *H. pylori.*

• Histamine-II receptor antagonist inhibits acid secretion.

• Antacids neutralize the gastric acid.

NB: Do not take milk as a treatment, as it stimulates acid secretion.

Complication

If the ulcer is bleeding, a person may develop anemia. In some cases perforation may complicate the ulcer.

Ulcers situated at the end part of the stomach where the duodenum is attached may cause swelling and obstruction of the duodenum. [xxxviii]

HEMORRHOIDS

Hemorrhoid is an enlargement of anorectal veins characterized by a painful swelling in the anorectal area. This condition is frequent to people who do not eat enough fiber and do suffer from constipation.

Symptoms

• Painful rectum and anus, especially on defecation.

• Hemorrhage may be present in some cases but not always.

• Mucus discharge.

• Irritation.

• Itching.

• Sensation of full rectum while it is empty.

NB: Constipation is not a symptom but a cause of hemorrhoid.

Causes

• Constipation

• Pregnancy

• Aging

• Heredity—there are people who inherit the weakness of anorectal veins wall from their parents.

Prevention

• Increase your intake of high-fiber food.

• Drink enough water.

• Avoid usage of laxatives.

• Avoid keeping stools for a long time in the rectum.

• Exercise to facilitate bowel movement.

Treatment

• Painkillers—but avoid those made with codeine, as it causes constipation.

• Eat a diet rich in fiber.

• Drink enough water.

• Avoid usage of laxatives.

• Avoid keeping stools for a long time in the rectum.

• Exercise to facilitate bowel movement.

• Consult your family doctor for medical attention.

• In some cases a surgical operation may be the solution. [xxxix]

TESTIS TORTION

Testis torsion is a condition characterized by a sudden and painful testis. The testis is reddish and hot. This may make the victim to be unable to walk properly.

It does happen mostly during puberty.

This condition is an extreme surgical emergency. The operation must be done within seventy-two hours from the time the pain started.

If the patient does not get help within seventy-two hours, necrosis will occur, and the person will lose his testis.

MENOPAUSE

Menopause is the cessation of the menstrual life.

There are three kinds of menopauses:

NATURAL MENOPAUSE

Natural menopause is due to age; this can be early, on time, or late.

PREMATURE MENOPAUSE

It is called premature menopause because it happens before the natural time of menopause. There are two different kinds of premature menopauses:

a. Chemical menopause: caused by certain drugs (ovary chemotherapy).
b. Surgical menopause: due to the removal of ovaries in a case of ovarian cancer.

COLD TURKEY MANOPAUSE

It is called cold turkey menopause when a woman is obliged to stop a hormonotherapy—for example, a woman takes estrogens because of menopausal side effects, and she develops breast cancer.

Side effects of menopauses

- Hot flushes

- Change of mood

- Osteoporosis—thin and fragile bones due to the lack of estrogens

- Dryness of the vagina (which affects sexual life)

- Insomnia

- Heart beating fast or tackycardia

- Hypertension

- Depression

How to prevent menopausal effects

- Eat a diet rich in minerals, vitamins and fibers (fruits, vegetables, seeds, whole grains, and legumes).

NB: Soy contains phytoestrogen, which is a natural ingredient that acts as an estrogen, but there is no proof that this will decrease hot flashes.

- Eat enough food rich in calcium and iron.

- Decrease saturated fat intake.

- Use sugar and salt moderately.

- Decrease alcohol intake but drink enough water.

- Exercise.

- Lose weight.

- Obtain hormone replacement if needed and if prescribed by a gynecologist.

- Get counseling.[xl]

HYPERTENSION

Hypertension is a persistent high arterial blood pressure, when the diastolic pressure (the second reading) is above 100 mm hg in a person over sixty years of age and ninety in a person under fifty years. In many cases hypertension is asymptomatic; that is why it is called a silent killer. But in some rare cases, a patient may present the following symptoms: Headaches, dizziness, sweating, and restlessness. There are two kinds of hypertension: primary and secondary.

PRIMARY HYPERTENSION

Primary or essential hypertension does not have an apparent cause, but it may be a consequence of emotional stress, anger, frustration, and resentment.

People with hypertension history in their families are at high risk of developing high blood pressure in their lifetimes. Primary hypertension is a permanent condition, but it may be very well controlled if treatment is taken as prescribed. The treatment is for life.

Risk factors of primary hypertension

• Age: hypertension risk increases with age.

• Sex: males are more exposed than females.

• Race: Blacks develop more hypertension than other races.

• History of hypertension in your family.

• Obesity: when you are overweight, you need more blood to supply oxygen and nutrients to your body cells, and when the amount of blood circulating in your body increases, it puts more pressure on your arteries' walls.

• Lack of exercise: People who do not exercise have a higher heart rate than those who do. The higher your heart rate is, the greater is your heart activity, and the more your heart works, the more your blood puts pressure on your arteries' walls.

• Salty diet: sodium increases fluids retention; the more you have fluid in your body, the more you predispose yourself to hypertension.

• Tobacco: it does damage your vessels lining; this may decrease the caliber of your vessels and cause hypertension.

• Alcohol: high consumption of alcohol may affect your heart and raise your blood pressure.

SECONDARY HYPERTENSION

Secondary hypertension is a consequence of some diseases. In this case hypertension is not a disease but a symptom and may totally disappear after the treatment of the cause.

Symptoms may be present or not, as is the case for primary hypertension.

Some conditions that may lead to hypertension

• Narrowing of one or both renal arteries

• Chronic glomerulonephritis (inflammation of some of the renal tissues)

• Pheochromocytoma (tumor of the middle part of the glands that are found on the upper part of kidneys and which produce an important amount of chemical that rise blood pressure)

• Coarctation of the aorta (constriction or stenosis of the aorta)

• Some medication like some contraceptives

• Primary hyperaldosteronism (high level of the hormone that is produced by a cortical part of the glands that are found on the upper part of the kidneys and which reabsorb sodium and rise blood pressure).

• Hyper/hypothyroidism

• Pregnancy: per example in a case of Preeclampsia (condition characterized by hypertension swollen legs and the presence of proteins in the urine during pregnancy).

• Stress

Complications of hypertension

High blood pressure may affect vessels and lead to atherosclerosis (destruction of the internal layer of arteries which promotes the accumulation of fats and obstruction). It may also cause the rupture of blood vessels and lead to stroke (brain), blindness (eye), or death (heart), according to the area of the affected vessel.

It may affect the eyes and lead to hypertensive retinopathy; it may affect the heart and lead to heart failure; it may affect kidneys and lead to kidney failure.

How do we prevent hypertension?

• Stop smoking.

• Decrease alcohol consumption.

• Avoid stress, and, if there is any, consult a professional for counseling. In some cases a medical consultation may be needed.

• Eat a diet low in sodium chloride but rich in fiber.

• Avoid saturated fats but take moderately low fat dairy products.

• Take food rich in potassium as it balances sodium level in your body cells,

• Add vitamin D in your diet as it affects aldosterone (hormone produced by the adrenal cortex and which causes retention of sodium and leads to hypertension),

• Exercise without competition.

• Lose weight if you are overweight.

• Regularly monitor your blood pressure to diagnose it early for good management.

What to do if diagnosed with hypertension

Consult your nearest clinic or your family doctor for assessment and management. The treatment is done in four stages:

• Weight loss

• A diet low in sodium chloride but rich in fiber and potassium

• Exercise

• Drugs

NB: Hypertension, being a chronic condition, is subject to treatment for life.[xli]

DIABETES MELLITUS

Diabetes mellitus is the insufficiency or lack of insulin secretion by the pancreas, characterized by a sugar metabolism disorder and manifested by a raised amount of sugar in the blood. This condition is permanent, but it may be very well managed if medication is taken as prescribed.

The treatment of diabetes mellitus is for life.

Symptoms

• Frequent urination

• Thirst

• Blurred vision

• Fatigue

• Paresthesia (burning, tickling, pricking sensation)

• Increase of appetite

Some patients are asymptomatic.

Causes

• Insufficient or lack of insulin secretion by the pancreas

• No response of body cells to insulin

There are two kinds of diabetes mellitus.

DIABETES MELLITUS TYPE 1

Diabetes mellitus type 1 is caused by total lack or diminution of pancreatic insulin secretion. This happens to young and non-obese patients.

Risk factors of diabetes type 1

• Genetic factors

• Some diseases of the pancreas

• Some infections or illnesses

DIABETES MELLITUS TYPE 2

Diabetes mellitus type 2 is caused by a non-response of body tissues to insulin. This happens to obese and older people.

Risk factors of diabetes type 2

• Obesity

• Genetic factors

• Hypertension

• Hyperlipidemia

•History of gestational diabetes

• Women who deliver fat babies over 4kg of weight at birth

• Lack of activity

• Polycystic ovaries syndrome

• Age over forty-five

Complications of diabetes mellitus

If diabetes mellitus is not well controlled, it may affect the eyes and lead to diabetic retinopathy. It may affect the heart, kidneys, skin, and nerves. It may affect lower limb vessels and lead to gangrene and amputation of the affected limb. Diabetes mellitus may lead to a coma and death.

How to prevent diabetes mellitus

1. Decrease your intake of food that gives energy, especially saturated fats and chemical sugar-rich foods, but eat enough high-fiber food.
2. Exercise regularly.
3. Lose weight.
4. Regular urine tests to diagnose it early for good management.

What to do if you are diagnosed with diabetes mellitus

• Avoid eating big amounts of food at the same time, but eat smaller portions on a regular basis.

• Decrease intake of foods that give energy (carbohydrates and fats), but increase your intake of high-fiber food.

• Decrease considerably the ingestion of chemical sugar.

• Avoid alcohol, soft drinks, and sweetened juice.

• Exercise regularly.

• Lose weight

• Take medication as prescribed by your physician, and respect the checkup appointments.[xlii]

ARTHRITIS

Arthritis is defined as an inflammation of joints.

There are three kinds of arthritis.

RHEUMATOID ARTHRITIS

Rheumatoid arthritis is defined as an autoimmune disease that may lead to a chronic inflammation of the fluid found within articulations (synovia) and can also affect several organs in a human body. The cause is not well known.

This disease may affect people at any age, but in most cases it starts between twenty and forty years of age. Females are more often affected than are males.

Risk factors

• Sex: females develop more rheumatoid arthritis than males.

• Age: it starts between twenty and forty years of age.

• Genetic factors.

• Smoking.

• It is also thought that some bacterial and viral infections may trigger the activation of the disease.

Symptoms

• Generalized malaise.

• Loss of weight.

• Periarticular stiffness and pain, with inflammation of tissues that surround the affected joint.

• Most of the time symptoms are acute and are caused by stress, emotion, infectious diseases, surgery, trauma, and post-partum conditions.

• The disease usually affects the articulations of fingers, wrists, knees, ankles, and toes.

• Synovial cyst and rupture of tendons may be present in complicated cases.

Prevention

Decrease the intake of saturated fats, as they contain a high level of arachidonic acid, which is a fatty acid that can be converted into prostaglandin (chemical responsible of inflammatory process in a human body), but increase your intake of high-fiber food.

Eat enough legumes, fruits, vegetables, and grains, as they are rich in phytonutrients (natural booster found in plants), antioxidants, and bioflavonoids (plant compound that have antiviral, anti-inflammatory, and anti-tumor properties).

Eat food rich in omega 3, as it contains eicosapentaenoic acid and docosahexaenoic acid. These have anti-inflammatory effects on a human body.

Exercise regularly. If you are obese, lose weight.

Treatment

The treatment in a case of rheumatoid arthritis is symptomatic.

The purpose of the treatment is to decrease inflammation, slow down or prevent joint damages, prevent disability, and to help a patient to maintain his mobility.

There are three lines in rheumatoid arthritis treatment:

1. Eat healthy, and lose weight if you overweight.

2. Exercise.

3. Use pain killers and anti inflammatory drugs.

Surgery may be needed in serious cases.

Please consult your nearest clinic or your family doctor for assessment and management.

Complications

The autoimmune process may affect the following:

- Articulations, causing stiffness

- The heart, and lead to pericardial effusion, or to myocarditis in some rare cases

- Blood vessels, and lead to the inflammation of blood vessels characterized by skin ulcers

- Lungs, and cause rheumatoid arthritis associated with interstitial lungs disease; rheumatoid arthritis pulmonary fibrosis; pleurisy; and lungs nodules.

- Eyes, and lead to inflammation of episclera that may lead to the loss of sight

- Skin, and lead to rheumatoid nodules

- Throat, and cause throat and vocal cords nodules, characterized by hoarseness of the voice

NB: Rheumatoid arthritis, when treated well from the early stage, is not dangerous and does not have serious complications.[xliii]

OSTEOARTHRITIS

Osteoarthritis is defined as a degenerative joint disease affecting people in their old age. In this kind of arthritis, there is degeneration of the connective tissues of an articulation, increase of bones' volume at the extremities, and changes in the articular membrane.

Symptoms

Symptoms include pains and stiffness, especially after physical activity.

Risk factors

- Old age

- Sex: females develop more osteoarthritis than males

- Congenital bones deformity and/or defective cartilage

- Joint injuries

- Obesity

- Lack of exercise

- Some diseases, such as diabetes, hypothyroidism, gout, and Paget's disease

Prevention

- Eat a diet rich in fiber, calcium, and magnesium: a daily tablet of calcium is recommended from age thirty-five.

- Exercise.

Treatment

- Lose weight.

- Avoid saturated fats and sugary foods, but increase your intake in high-fiber food (fruits, legumes, and vegetables).

- Avoid food cooked at high temperatures, as that produces

an advanced glycation end product, which may lead to inflammatory processes in the body and may contribute to the activation of some other diseases, such rheumatoid arthritis, heart disease, nephropathy, and diabetes.

- Drink enough water meaning two liters per day for an adult.

- Eat food rich in omega 3 (fish like Salmon and Tuna) or take a supplement; omega 3 decreases the morning stiffness associated with osteoarthritis.

- Use olive oil instead of other oils. It is rich in oleochanthal (a natural anti-inflammatory compound). It works in the same way as NSAIDs. A serving of 35 ml (three-and-a-half tablespoons) gives the same pain-relief result as 200 mgs of ibuprofen.

- Increase your intake of food rich in vitamin C (lemon, oranges). It helps to build up collagen and connective tissues.

- Take a supplement of glucosamine sulfate 1500mg per day and chondroitin 800-1000mg per day. This may decrease pain and improve mobility to some people.

NB: Some supplements may interact with some medication.

- Please consult your nearest clinic or family doctor for management.

- Surgery may be the solution in serious cases (Joint replacement)

Complications

The complications of osteoarthritis are pain and limitation of activities.[xliv]

GOUT

Gout is a chronic hereditary metabolic disease characterized by an increase of uric acid in the blood. This uric acid deposits in and around peripheral joints. The increase of uric acid may be caused by an increased rate of synthesis of uric acid or by the kidney's decrease of elimination of uric acid, or it may be both.

Causes

Genetic factors are the cause of gout.

Risk factors

You are at a high risk of developing gout when the level of uric acid in your blood is high. Here are some factors that increase the level of uric acid in the blood:

• Obesity.

• Hypertension.

• Diabetes mellitus.

• Hyperlipidemia and atherosclerosis.

• Leukemia, lymphoma.

• Hemoglobin disorder.

• Certain drugs, such as hydrochlorothiazide, pyrazinamide, cyclosporine, niacin, aspirin, ethambutol, anti-rejection drugs (prescribed to people who underwent organ transplant).

• Alcohol, as it may cause dehydration, which is one of the causes of acute gout attack. Alcohol may also affect uric acid metabolism and lead to hyperuricemia.

• Food rich in purine, such as the following:

Red meat

Animal organs (e.g., liver, kidneys, brains)

Shellfish

Sweetbreads

Fructose from corn syrup found in some cold drinks

NB: The body converts purine into uric acid. Some factors (e.g., fever, dehydration, alcohol intake, excessive eating, and recent surgery) may precipitate an acute gout attack.

Symptoms

All the symptoms of acute arthritis are present, but in this case only one peripheral joint is affected at once.

Prevention

Eliminate all the above risk factors to prevent gout.

Treatment

• Diet: Avoid eating food rich in purine, but eat enough high-fiber food.

• Drink a lot of water (at least two liters per day for an adult).

• Decrease alcohol consumption.

• Exercise.

• Lose weight.

• Consult your doctor for medical treatment.

Complications

• Recurrent gout.

• Tophi—this happens in advanced gout, when deposits of urate crystals form nodules under the skin.

Kidney stones.[xlv]

PROSTITIS

For you to understand prostitis, you have first to know what the prostate is. The prostate is a male gland that produces 20 to 30 percent of the volume of semen and spermatozoids.

Prostitis is an infection of the prostate; most of the time it is associated with lower urinary-tract infection. The germs causing the infection may reach the prostate via blood circulation (when there is infection somewhere else inside the body).

Symptoms

- Hesitancy on initiating urination, caused by the compression of the urethra by an inflamed prostate

- Pains on the part between the anus and the testis as well as behind the anus.

- Fever

- Urethral discharge

- Lower spinal-cord pain

Complications

- Inflammation of bladder and testis

- Inflammation and obstruction of urethra

- Urinary tract infection

- Urinary retention

Treatment

- Antibiotics.
- Painkillers.
- Diet rich in fibers.
- Drink enough water, but little by little.

- Exercise.

- Prostate massage.[xlvi]

PROSTATISME

Prostatism is a syndrome happening to some males age fifty and older, caused by the change in the nature of prostate cells, which become hard due to age and are characterized by the enlargement of the gland.

NB: A blood test: prostate serum antigen (PSA) must be done on a regular basis to exclude any malignancy.

Symptoms

- Frequent and urgent urination, especially during the night.

- Releases only a small amount of urine at once but on a regular basis

- Urine hesitancy

- Decrease of urinary caliber and stream

- Urinary retention

- Painful urination

- Painful ejaculation

- Bloody semen

- Sexual dysfunction

- Recurrent urinary tract infection

Complications

- Urinary retention

- Urinary tract infection

- Bladder stones

- Decompensate bladder

Medical treatment

The doctor will start by treating the infection, if any, and supplying painkillers and muscle relaxants; in serious cases, surgery may be necessary.

Natural treatment

- Eat a diet rich in fiber.

- Drink enough water but little by little.

- Avoid sugar, caffeine, dairy products, fried food, junk food, and refined food.

- Exercise of the prostate (keeping your muscles in your stomach and strengthening them will increase blood flow of all the organs in your stomach). This will help you to feel better.

- Massage of the prostate improve blood flow in the prostate and decrease pain.

- Prostate's drainage (insertion of a finger in the rectum on a regular basis with a purpose of increasing the pressure on the prostate).

- Frequent ejaculation (at least two to three times a week)
- Sitz Baths: sitting in hot water for more than twenty minutes alleviate the pain.

Natural supplements

1.Zinc: thirty milligrams of zinc per day maintain the prostate and prevent infections.

2.Licopen and betacaroten found in tomatoes decrease the risk of developing prostate cancer.

3.Vitamin C (500-1000mg per day) and E (400 IUs per day) decrease the inflammatory process and prevent prostate cancer.

4.Selenium as an antioxidant prevent the oxidation and inflammatory process in the prostate gland.

5.Proteilytic enzyme has an anti-inflammatory property

6.Magnesium supplement maintain   the prostate and decrease   the risk of prostatisme.

7. Bromelain 400 mg three times per day

8. Flaxseed meal: two to four tablespoons per day, it is rich in fibers and vitamins.

8.Goldenseal is a diuretic and antimicrobial

9.Corn silk is a natural diuretic

10.Cornflower improves the immune system

11.Uva ursi, used as natural diuretic and urinary antiseptic.

12.Echinacea (natural booster found in plants)

13.Saw palmetto is a plant used to treat symptoms of an enlarged prostate

14. Bearberry acts as a diuretic and antiseptic for the urinary tract

15. Flower pollen extract decrease the pain.[xlvii]

ANTIBIOTHERAPY

Antibiotherapy is a treatment using antibiotics. Antibiotics are substances that inhibit the growth of bacteria or kill them.

There are several antibiotics families and among the same family several groups.

When an individual takes antibiotics, the most sensitive germs will die from the first day, but the stronger ones may die only on the last day of the treatment. Antibiotics must be prescribed only by a medical practitioner and must be taken as prescribed. The strength, the number of times per day, the interval between the intakes of a specific antibiotic, and the number of days must be respected. For example, if a doctor prescribes 500 mgs of amoxicillin three times per day for seven days, she means it, and it must be so. Some people mistakenly stop taking their antibiotic treatment once they feel better; others decrease either the strength per intake, or the number of daily intakes and others do both. This must not be an option.

When you do not take your antibiotics properly, that will work against you; it will do to the germs what a vaccine does to your body, because germs will develop resistance to that specific antibiotic, and they will transmit that genetic material of that drug's resistance to the next generation of germs.

This means that specific antibiotic may not help you properly in the future.

NB: This process is the same for all antimicrobials (antibiotics, antivirus, and antifungal drugs).

GUIDELINES WHEN YOU ARE CONSULTING ANY MEDICAL INSTITUTION OR ANY MEDICAL PRACTITIONER

• Take along all the drugs you are taking and show your doctor, so he may know what else to prescribe for you, as there are medicines that must not be taken together.

• Remember to tell your doctor about a pre-existing disease or condition, if any.

Let your doctor know that you are pregnant or breastfeeding. Talk to her about your allergies and if you are allergic to anything.

NB: Remember your doctor is a suitable person of whom you may ask any questions concerning your condition.

• Follow very well your doctor's instructions.

• Before you leave your doctor's office, ask him which one among the prescribed medicines is an antimicrobial.

NB: Never forget that all antimicrobials (antibiotics, antiviral, and antifungal) must be taken properly until the last drop.

CONCLUSION

We must always visit our clinics and family doctors without delay once we notice some abnormal signs in our bodies. We must not wait for the time we are too sick to consult, as it may be too late.

There are diseases that show symptoms from early stages, but others may show symptoms only when it is already late. That is why it is recommended that everybody, men and women, do general checkups at least once a year. This means a blood test to check the following:

• Whether the kidneys function well and to detect early kidney failure.

• Liver function to diagnose the status of the liver.

• Cholesterol level.

• Women must once a year have a mammogram, to detect the beginning of breast cancer, and a pap smear, to detect the beginning of cervical cancer.

• Men need to check PSA (prostate serum antigen) from age forty and once they notice a blockage of urine.

• Blood pressure monitoring and urine test to detect diabetes mellitus may be done every month.

• Routine eye examination must be done every two years.

• Consult your dentist every six months.

[i] *Stedman's Medical dictionary for the Health Professions and Nursing, illustrated* 5th edition, page 641

[ii] *Stedman's Medical Dictionary for the Health Professions and Nursing, illustrated* 5th edition, page 1215

[iii] Pam Belluck, Boys Now Enter Puberty Younger, Study Suggests, but It's Unclear Why, October 20, 2012, www.nytimes.com/2012/10/20/health/p...read on the 12 July 2013.

[iv] *Dorland Illustrated Medical Dictionary*, 25th edition, page 42

[v] Marcus A.Krupp, and Milton A Chatton, *Current Medical Diagnosis and Treatment* (1979), New York: Large Medical Publications, 808. 905

[vi] WebMD, Food and recipes, protein: Are You Getting Enough? www.webmd.com/food-recipes/protein

[vii] Center for Diseases Control and Prevention, "Nutrition for Everyone: Vitamins and Minerals"

[viii] www.cdc.gov: Centers for Disease Control and Prevention: Nutrition for everyone, vitamins and minerals, 23 Feb 2011. www.ods.od.nih.gov: Office of Dietary Supplements: Vitamins and mineral supplement fact sheets, general supplement information.

www.webMD.com: WebMD Food source for vitamins and minerals. Australian government, Department of Health and Ageing, vitamin and minerals, 20 Jul 2006.

[ix] www.healthch ecksystems.com/antioxidants
www.wikipedia.org/wiki/radical (chemistry)
www.wisegeek.org/ What are free radicals? 24 Feb 2013.

[x] Health Check System, Understanding Free Radicals and Antioxidants: //www.heathchecksystems.com/antioxid.htm
[xi] WebMD, "The benefits of fiber: For your heart, weight, and energy, Dietary fiber: Insoluble vs. Soluble."

[xii] www.webmd.com/diet/fiber-health-benefit
www.wikipedia.org/wiki/Dietary fiber
www.wildfibersmagazine.com

[xiii] Official Partner of the Livestrong Foundation, what is a serving size in grams of protein, Sept 28, 2010 by James Roland, read on 12 Jul 2013
[xiv] Marcus A. Krupp, and Milton A. Chatton, *Current Medical Diagnosis and Treatment* (1979), New York: Lange Medical Publications, page 809.

[xv] Marcus A.Krupp, and Milton A Chatton, *Current Medical Diagnosis and Treatment* (1979), New York: Large Medical Publications, page 808.
[xvi] www.wikipedia.org/wiki/avitaminosis
www.thefreedictionary.com/avitaminosis
www.rightdiagnosis.com>Diseases> avitaminosis, 1 Mar 2013.

[xvii] Greg Amold,DC,CSCS, Omega 3 Fats,Vitamin C and EHelp Pancreas Health, found at
www.now.university.com>Home>Library>Nutrients>Omega.3Fa
tty Acids, September 27, 2010

[xviii] *Dorland Illustrated Medical Dictionary*, 25th edition, page 1064

[xix] *Stedman's Medical Dictionary for the Health Professions and Nursing illustrated* 5th edition, page 695

[xx] About.com cholesterol, the dangers of high cholesterol and diabetes [add URL/web address]

[xxi] American Heart Association, Hypertension, circulation, atherosclerosis.
www.wikipedia.org/wiki/endothelium
www.wikipedia.org/wiki/Low-density lipoprotein
www.webmd.com/cholesterol/managment
www.mayoclinic.com>home> diseases and conditions>high cholesterol
www.wikipedia.org/wiki/cholesterol
MedilinePlus, Cholesterol.
NIH, National Heart, Lung, and Blood Institute, What is cholesterol?
www.nhlbi.nih.gov>home>Health information for the public>Health topics
www.cholesterol.about.com

[xxi] Mayo clinic, high cholesterol

[xxii] Centers for Disease Control and Prevention, Diseases and conditions, seasonal flu, about flu.
Marcus A. Krupp and Milton J. Chatton, page 837.
Centers for Disease Control and Prevention, For everyone: Preventing seasonal flu illness.
WebMD, Cold, Flu and Cough Health Center.
www.wikipedia.org/wiki/influenza

[xxiiixxiii] South African Department of Health, *Standard Treatment Guidelines and Essential Drugs List*, 2008 edition, page 267.

[xxiv] South African Department of Health, *Standard treatment guidelines and essential drugs list*, 2008 edition, page 267.

Marcus A. Krupp and Milton J. Chatton, pages *Current medical diagnostic and treatment* 1979, paes:119–122.
WebMD, Asthma Health Center.
www.asthma.org.UK

www.medicalnewstoday.com>Home>respiratory/asthma
[xxv] Mims, *Diseases Review* 3003, *Antimicrobial*/infectious diseases.
NHS Choices, Tonsillitis.
Marcus A. Krupp and Milton J. Chatton *Current medical diagnostic and treatment* 1979, pages 108–109.
www.webmd.com/oral-health/guide/tonsillitis
www.patient.co.uk, Tonsillitis.

[xxvi] www.webmd.com/allergies-sinusitis
National Institute of Allergy and Infectious Diseases, Sinusitis.
www.patient.co.uk,acute sinusitis
Marcus A. Krupp and Milton J. Chatton, *Current medical diagnosis and treatment* 1979, pages 106 –107.

[xxvii] MedlinePlus, otitis.
www.wikipedia.org/wiki/otitis
Marcus A. Krupp and Milton J. Chatton, *Current medical diagnostic and treatment* 1979, papages 100–101.
Centers for Disease Control and Prevention, Ear infections.

[xxviii] www.webmd.com/epilepsy
www.epilepsy.com
NHS choices, epilepsy.
Marcus A. Krupp and Milton J. Chatton, pages *Current medical diagnostic and treatment* 1979, paes:594–599.

[xxix] www.kidsHealth,org from Nmours, all about puberty
TeensHealth, Everything you wanted to know about puberty.

[xxx] Krupp and Chatton , pages 657

[xxxi] Stedman's, page 931

[xxxii] Ibid, page 1181

[xxxiii] www.masminaturalcotton.com: vulvo-vaginal irritation.
Krupp and Chatton , pages 453–457.
Medscape, Omnia M. Samra, Vulvo-vaginitis, 13 Jan 2012.

[xxxiv] www.wikipedia.org/wiki/candidiasis
Netdoctor, Dr. Roger Henderson, Vaginal thrush (candidiasis), 20 Sept 2011.
MedlinePlus, Vaginal yeast infection.
Krupp and Chatton, page 457.

[xxxv] Krupp and Chatton, page 425

[xxxvi] Krupp and Chatton, page 459

[xxxvii] Krupp and Chatton, page 461

[xxxviii] Brunner and Suddarth's, Suzanne C. Smeltzer, Brenda Bare, *Medical Surgical Nursing* 10th edition, pages 1015–1027.
WebMD, Digestive Disorder Health Center, What is peptic ulcer disease?
MedicineNet.com, Peptic ulcer disease.
Krupp and Chatton, pages 366–369.

[xxxix] Brunner and Suddarth's, pages 1066–1067.
Mayo clinic, Diseases and conditions, Hemorrhoids.
Krupp and Chatton, page 393.
www.emedicinehealth.com,hemorrhoids
WebMD, Hemorrhoids, 22 Sept 2010.

[xl] www..wikipedia.org/wiki/menopause
Mayo Clinic, Menopause.
WebMD, Menopause health center.
www.womenshealth,gov, Menopause.
www.healthBoards.com Menopause.

[xli] Brunner and Suddarth's, pages 855–866.
Krupp and Chatton, pages 191–192 and 729–730.

Meena S. Madhur, MD, PhD, Hypertension, 4 Feb 2013.

[xlii] Brunner and Suddarth's, pages 1150–1203.
www.wikipedia.org/wiki/diabetes mellitus
Krupp and Chatton, pages 759–772.
WebMD, Diabetes health center, Types of diabetes mellitus.
[xliii] WebMD, Rheumatoid arthritis health center, Rheumatoid
arthritis (RA) complications.
University of Maryland Medical Center, Rheumatoid arthritis.
Krupp and Chatton, pages 506–512.
WebMD, Rheumatoid arthritis health center, Can your diet help
relieve rheumatoid arthritis?
Katherine K. Temprano, MD, Rheumatoid arthritis, 2 Feb 2013.
www.wikipedia.org/wiki/eicosapentaenoic acid
www.rheumatology.oxfordjournals.org/com
www.wikipedia.org/wiki/arachidonic acid

[xliv] Marcus A. Krupp and Milton J. Chatton, pages 522–523.
Carlos Lozada, MD, Osteoarthritis, 22 Jan 2013.
www.wikipedia.org/wiki/osteoarthritis
www.wikipedia.org/wiki/advanced glycation end product
www.ncbi.nim.nih.gov/pubmed/advanced glycation end products
www.sparkpeople.com>nutrition article> special concerns:
Time for wellness, olive oil more effective than medical gel.
Arthritis, Glucosamine and Chondroitin,
www.arthritisvic.org.au>Home>Complementary Therapies, 12
July 2013.

[xlv]Marcus A. Krupp and Milton J. Chatton, *Current medical
diagnostic and treatment* 1979, pages 526–530.
Bruce M Rothschild, MD, Gout and pseudogout, 09 Jan 2013.
www.wikipedia.org/wiki/gout
WebMD, Arthritis health center, Gout topic overview: what is
gout?
[xlvi] Mayo Clinic, prostitis.
www.wikipedia.org/wiki/prostitis

[xlvii] BBC health, Dr. Rob Hicks, prostatism
WebMD, Health news, Sid Kirchheimer, Prostate cancer health
center, 04 Feb 2003.
www.seacoast.com: Prostatism natural treatment
Marcus A. Krupp and Chatton, *Current medical diagnostic and treatment* 1979, page 583.
La prostate, votre santé par la nature,
santenature.over.blog.com/article.i, 12 July 2013
Steady health.com, how to treat prostatitis with natural
supplements? By Dr Herold Gladwell, May 3, 2007